LCE

LEARN CARE EXCEL

WWW.LEARNCAREEXCEL.CO.UK

Mental Capacity & Deprivation of Liberty In Care Course Book

OTHER PUBLICATIONS IN THE SERIES:

Nutrition in the Care Setting (01NCS)
Food Hygiene (02FH)
Fire Safety (03FS)
Safeguarding Vulnerable Adults (04SV)
End of Life Care, Death and Bereavement (05DB)
Person-Centred Planning (06PC)
Diabetes (07DD)
Stroke (08SS)
Dementia Care (09DC)
Managing Aggression (10MA)
Mental Health Issues (11MH)
Health and Safety (12HS)
Medication (13MM)
Infection Control (14IC)
Equality and Inclusion (15EI)

For information on this or other courses please contact:

LEARN CARE EXCEL

Matthews House
21 Thorley Park Road
Bishops Stortford
CM23 3NG

Tel: 07774 880880

info@learncareexcel.co.uk
www.learncareexcel.co.uk

Contents

INTRODUCTION

Most of us take for granted the right and ability to make decisions for ourselves and move around as we choose but there are certain limited situations in which people can no longer do this. Just because we lose our ability, however, to take a decision for ourselves does not mean that we lose all our rights in the decision making process and there are several laws that protect a person when they are in a vulnerable position.

A person's ability to make a decision or to be safe left on their own varies from person to person, from time to time and from situation to situation. A ten year old child, for instance is perfectly capable of deciding what flavour ice cream they would like to have but not to know who is safe to befriend on social media. This is why the lower age limit on Facebook is 16. Equally, a person with learning difficulty may be well aware of needing to save money to buy an expensive piece of jewellery but may not fully grasp the necessity to save for their retirement. Finally an elderly person may still have a very active and shrewd mind when it comes to day to day decision but changes in their medical condition may mean that they need to be on medication which affects the way they think.

People working in the care industry must be particularly aware that the people that they look after, purely by virtue of the fact that they are "looked after", are vulnerable and hence there is a moral imperative and legal obligation to preserve their rights, in the same way that they care for their physical health and wellbeing.

There are several laws which protect vulnerable people in this case including the Mental Capacity Act 2005, the Human Rights Act 1998 and the Equality Act 2010. But the key thing to remember is that everyone has the right to make decisions for themselves, or be involved in the decision making process, to as much an extent as is possible and simply making a bad decision is not proof that they should have that right taken away.

As with all the texts in this series, information in this course book is aimed at workers in the care industry and discussion will concentrate particularly on the effects and treatment of the adults in these settings. If you are supporting younger people or people with specific needs please consult further texts.

WHAT IS MENTAL CAPACITY?

Simply put, "mental capacity" is the ability to rationally figure out how to do something. In terms of the law, however, mental capacity is the standard by which someone is deemed able to make their own decisions in a specific situation. It is expected that everyone should be treated as though they have the capacity to make their own decisions unless it has been proven that they cannot. It also means that there may be varying degrees to which someone can become involved in the decisions made for them, even if they are not able to make the entire decision alone.

THE LAW AND MENTAL CAPACITY

At this point it important to look at the key Acts which affect how vulnerable people are treated when it comes to their rights. The first of these is the Mental Capacity Act:

MENTAL CAPACITY ACT 2005

This Act was fully implemented in 2007 and replaced part 7 of the Mental Health Act 1983. This also replaced the ENDURING POWER Of ATTORNEY ACT 1985.

This Act offers guidance as to how to treat people who can make some decisions about their treatment, and live a mainly independent life, but who may need help with some other aspects of their life – such as being able to live independently but needing help to cook hot meals.

This Act also incorporates the principle of 'advanced decisions' which is when someone with suitable mental capacity decides that they do not want a particular type of treatment if they lack capacity in the future to decide or to express this decision. A doctor must respect this decision.

Finally, this Act criminalized neglect meaning that a person accused of neglecting another is breaking the law and can be dealt with through the criminal justice system.

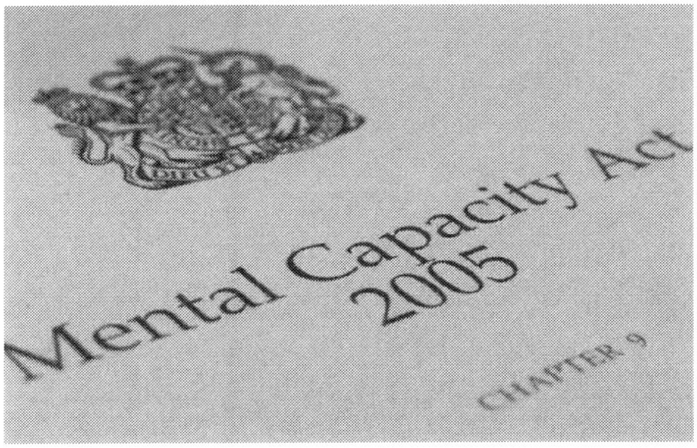

THE MENTAL HEALTH ACT 1983

This is the Act which made it possible to, in certain very strict circumstances, to detain someone against their wishes if it is in the best interest of themselves or the public at large. This is known as Deprivation of Liberty.

Most people with mental health issues receive their treatment and carry on with their normal lives while in the community. Some people, however, can experience severe mental health problems that require admission to hospital for assessment and treatment. Again, most of those will go in to hospital voluntarily with the hope that it will help them to improve. Some of these people do not wish to admit that they need to be hospitalised, or are too ill to realise the severity of their problem, and these people need to be held against their will. To avoid abuse of this power, however, people can only be detained if the strict criteria laid down in the Act are met:

- The person must be suffering from a mental disorder as defined by the Act.
- An application for assessment or treatment must be supported in writing by two registered medical practitioners.
- The recommendation must include a statement about why an assessment and treatment is necessary, including why other methods of dealing with the patient are not appropriate.

In addition to the Acts specifically relating to mental capacity there are other Acts which work alongside them such as the:

HUMAN RIGHTS ACT 1998 which enshrines into UK law the fundamental rights and freedoms contained in the European Convention on Human Rights and the Universal Declaration of Human Rights from the United Nations. These rights not only impact matters of life and death, they also affect the rights of everyday life: what a person can say and do, what beliefs they may hold, the right to a fair trial and other similar basic entitlements.

Everyone has the responsibility to respect and preserve other people's rights. When it comes to someone's mental capacity the following rights specifically apply:

- freedom from torture and degrading treatment
- the right to liberty
- the right to a fair trial
- the right to respect for private and family life
- freedom of thought, conscience and religion, and freedom to express your beliefs
- freedom of expression
- the right not to be discriminated against in respect of these rights and freedoms

Most rights have limits to ensure that they do not unfairly affect other people's rights, including our own.

EQUALITY ACT 2010 aims to eliminate unlawful discrimination, harassment and victimisation, promote fairness, equality opportunity and good relations, and create a legal requirement that people and places of work protect themselves and others from discrimination. This Act joined together all the previous legislation surrounding discrimination including:

- Disability Discrimination Act 1995
- Race Relations (Amendment) Act 2000
- Sex Discrimination Act 1975
- Employment Equality (Age) Regs 2006
- Employment Equality (Religion or Belief) Regs 2003
- Employment Equality (Sexual Orientation) Regs 2003
- Equal Pay Act 1970 Equality Act 2005 Act which amended or extended existing provisions in the DDA 1995 including ensuring that discrimination law covers all the activities of the public sector and that these bodies should actively promote equality of opportunity for disabled people

There are two key methods the Equality Act employs to achieve its aim:

1. **Protected Groups** - The Act also sets out "protected groups" in order to make it clear who is at risk of discrimination and who needs extra consideration. There are currently nine Protected Characteristics under the Equality Act 2010. These are:

Age	Disability	Race
Gender	Sexual Orientation	Gender reassignment
Religion and Belief	Marriage and Civil Partnership	Pregnancy and Maternity

2. **Protection for Whistle Blowers** - In addition to setting up enforceable laws which will lead to punishment if they are breached, the Act encourages vigilance for illegal or unfair acts as well as offering support for people who come forward to report these incidents.

REMEMBER

Ignorance of the law is no excuse!

Discrimination against a service user is abuse and, because of the extra duty of care, is taken more seriously and hence will be reported to SOVA

It may not be just an employer, but could also be a colleague, a client or someone else. It may be one significant event or repeated, low-level treatment intended to undermine

REPORT IT!

If someone witnesses or is a victim of discrimination, harassment or victimisation and the employer does nothing about it, they are complicit and become part of the problem.

More information on these laws can be found in our *Equality and Inclusion (15EI)* text book.

HOW DO THESE ACTS WORK TOGETHER TO PROTECT THE VULNERABLE?

Following best practice these Acts work together in the following key ways to offer clear guidance for carers and professionals about when someone is mentally capable of making their own decisions:

It's the Law:

First of all, it makes it a legal requirement to establish that someone's mental fitness before taking away their right to make a decision and then treat them fairly and without prejudice, with any infringement potentially punishable by reprimand, dismissal, a fine and even imprisonment. It is the responsibility of everyone to understand and actively carry out the laws and respect each other's rights and under the law ignorance is no excuse.

It Enhances the Moral Imperative:

Rather than concentrating on the punitive aspect of why the Acts should be followed it is helpful to consider the positive aspects. Work places that exhibit a strong ethos of following the law in relation to mental capacity and respecting each other's rights as individuals benefit from trust, flexibility, a motivated workforce and people feeling valued and respected, to name a few.

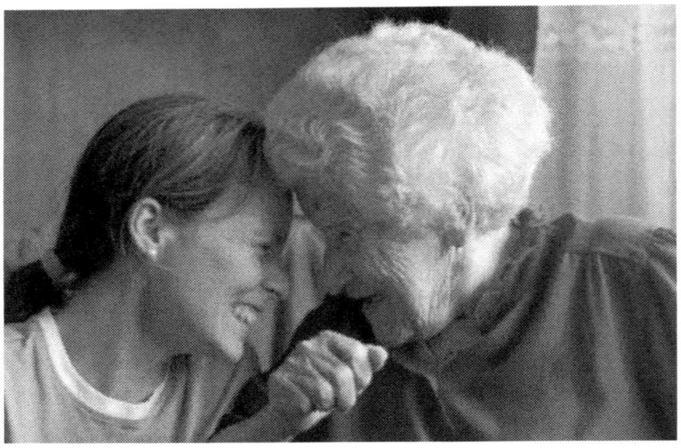

There are many reasons a person's ability to make a decision is impaired (including learning difficulty, dementia or depression) and, as people's ability can vary over time or with the difficulty of the issue, and, as decisions can vary in their complexity or gravity, under the Act a person's ability to make a decision must be judged on a case by case basis.

Generally, however, a person is considered able to make a decision unless one of the following can be proven:

- They are unable to understand the information given to them
- They are unable to retain this information long enough to consider the decision
- They are unable to consider and use this information as part of a rational decision making process
- They are unable to communicate their decision in an understandable way (this does not have to be verbally and could even just be a blink)

There are many reasons that a person may not be able to make a decision but workers in the care industry should be conscious that they may come across more people in these situations than other industries. For instance, carers will deal with a higher proportion than average of people with dementia or those recovering from a stroke. Due to the fact that residents are often disoriented when they move to a home they may feel confused or overwhelmed or people may be on medication that affects their ability to reason. And these are in addition to all of the factors that affect people outside the care industry such as mental health problems like schizophrenia, learning difficulties and drug or alcohol misuse.

Accordingly there may be times when, if a decision is not urgent, there should be a delay until the person is better able to understand the information, consider the options and communicate their wishes. For instance, someone suffering from diabetes may become incoherent if they become hypoglycaemic but this is a temporary situation so any decision should be postponed until their diabetes has been brought under control again.

We all have times when making a decision is difficult and we all make bad decisions occasionally but this does not mean we do not have the capacity to decide. One or more of the above must be proven before anyone can take away someone's right to make a decision.

REMEMBER

Lack of capacity to make a decision can vary over time and in relation to complexity.
The right to decide should be considered on a case by case basis.

Once it has been established that someone cannot be left to make a decision unaided there are certain procedures which must be followed. Under the Mental Health Act 2005 there are 5 principles to follow when supporting a person to make a decision. These are known as the Five Principles and they form the fundamental central theme of the Act:

5 PRINCIPLES

PRINCIPLE 1 An individual presumed to have capacity until it is proven that they do not.

PRINCIPLE 2 An individual should be supported to make their own decisions.

PRINCIPLE 3 A person should not be treated as unable to make a decision because they make an unwise decision.

PRINCIPLE 4 A decision made under the act has to be done so in the persons ‘best interests’.

PRINCIPLE 5 Before a person’s rights are overridden thought must be given as to how this can be done in the least restrictive way possible.

In order to comply with these principles the following advice can be used:

- Give clear information about the choices that are available to them.
- Ensure information is given in context (e.g in the setting where the activity will be).
- Arrange the environment in a way that helps better communication.
- Choose a time when they are more receptive (when they are more lucid)
- Give the information in a way that the person can understand.
- Monitor their response, and get feedback on what is happening to gauge their understanding.

The aim of these principles is to empower and protect people whose capability to make decisions is reduced. They provide a framework through which a person can be supported in their decision making as well as a system for settling disputes, dealing with personal welfare and managing their property and affairs. And this framework can be applied to the big decisions (such as whether to attempt resuscitation if the individual dies) and small (such as whether they would like sugar in their tea).

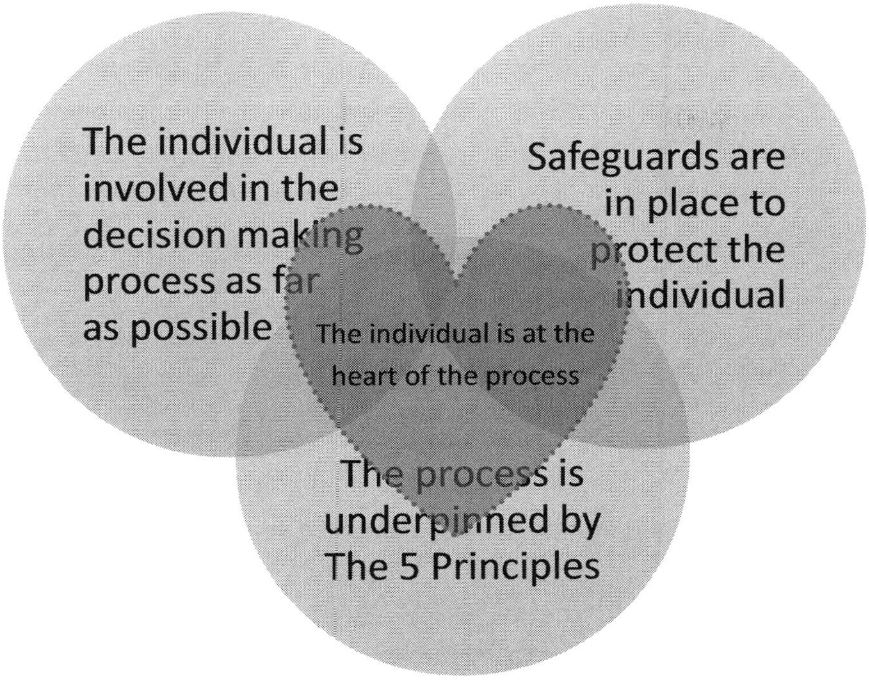

Code of Practice

Through following the tests for capability and The 5 Principles a Code of Practice has been established to assist the people who are assisting those who are vulnerable. This means that:

- There is a clear test for establishing capability
- There are clear parameters for determining what is in a person's best interest
- Individuals remain able to contribute to the decision making process wherever possible
- There is clear guidance on what actions may be taken on behalf of someone
- There are clear safeguards to protect the individual from discrimination or abuse
- Wilful neglect or ill-treatment of those requiring assistance is an offence under the law
- There is an obligation to consult with anyone interested in the welfare of the individual if they require assistance with their decision making
- Independent advocacy is available under the law for individuals requiring assistance and the Court of Protection or Office of Public Guardian may appoint a Public Guardian to protect the interests of the individual who requires assistance.

The aim is to protect the person with reduced capacity, not run their life for them!

When considering whether someone needs assistance in their decision making the very first thing to do is to assess their capability. This can be done following the test as laid out the Act (discussed above) but there are several things to consider when assessing someone's capacity.

First and foremost an assessment must start from the assumption that the person IS mentally capable. This is because an assessment of mental capability is done on a case by case, decision by decision, basis. Just because someone needed assistance with the previous decision does not necessarily mean that they will require assistance with the current one.

It is a requirement under the MCA that an assessment of mental capacity is carried out whenever a decision needs to be made about care arrangements or medical treatment. Significantly, the more serious the decision the more formal the assessment will need to be, including the recording of the process of assessment and the decision.

The above requirement, however, does not mean that this is the only time an assessment will need to be done, just every time a decision of that nature needs to be made. When it comes to other decisions throughout the day to day lives of vulnerable people the carer will need to use their judgement and experience as to how deeply, if at all, an assessment will be required.

Assessments must be "decision specific"

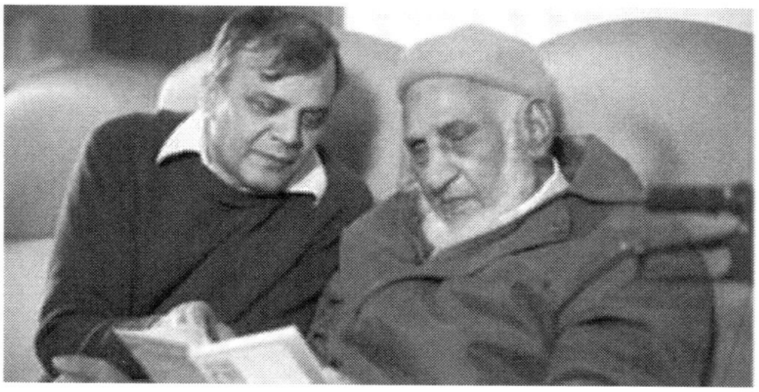

ASSESSING THE FUNCTIONAL IMPACT OF AN IMPAIRED CAPACITY

Once it has been established that someone may have an impaired capacity the next thing to understand to what extent that impairment, if any, will affect their ability to make the current decision. This is called a test of "functionality"

It may be that the person is not able to understand the implications of their situation (such as someone suffering from dementia) or it may be that they are not able to go through a rational decision making process (such as someone with learning difficulties) or it may mean that they are not able to communicate their decision (such as someone who has had a stroke).

Depending on the situation there may be a need to help the person understand the information (for instance writing it down rather than telling them) or it may mean that they need assistance understanding (when the carer can take some extra time to explain the implications) or the carer may need to find other ways to understand the person's instructions (such as asking for them to squeeze their hand).

Occasionally the assessment of the care staff will be challenged by the person who has been assessed or someone acting for them. In these cases an examination of the records relating to the assessment can be helpful to understand the background to the assessment. If this does not resolve the situation then it may be advisable to get a second opinion. If neither of these resolve the issue then there is recourse via the home's complaints procedures, mediation, a case conference with local social service agencies or, in the most extreme cases, seek a ruling from the Court of Protection.

Don't influence a decision by expressing your own opinion!

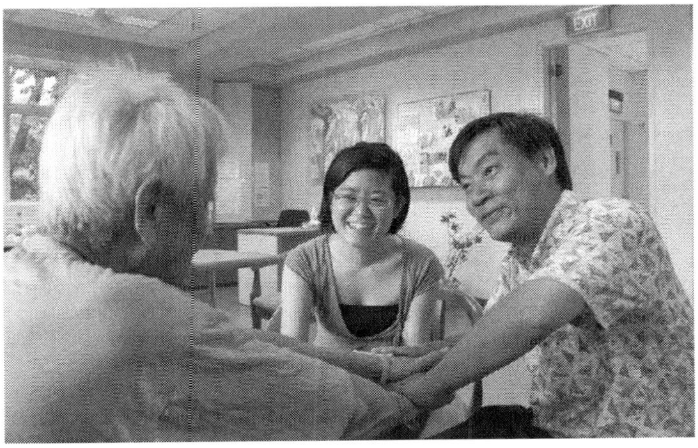

It may be the case that the carer is not able to adequately enable the person to make their decision completely on their own, in which case there will have to be a decision made on behalf of the individual, but in the best interests of that individual.

"Decision makers" are people who make decisions on behalf of individuals who cannot and include people such as carers who are in charge of the day to day care of the person, medical professionals such as a GP, family member of the person, or an independent person who has been appointed to the role. Where a dispute arises the same guidelines apply as the assessment process.

Sometimes there will be no need to involve others and the carer can act alone but this will only relate to simple decisions which will have no impact on the wellbeing of the individual. For instance, if the person has had a stroke and cannot communicate, the carer could decide to add sugar to their tea on behalf of the individual because that is how they always had it before the stroke. Actually, the stroke may have affected the centre of the brain which affects the person's taste and they would now prefer to have it without but in the absence of any evidence to the contrary the carer will have made their best judgement and, even if it is wrong, the implications are minimal.

There are several key points to remember when making proper decisions on behalf of someone else:

- ✓ Do involve the individual as much as possible in the decision making process, including taking into account their past preferences, any written down wishes, and any beliefs and values that would affect the decision
- ✓ Do consult other people before making a decision on behalf of a vulnerable person such as a relative of the person, someone the person named before the reduction in their capacity or an appointed court official. In the case of serious medical decisions the services of an Independent Mental Capacity Advocate (IMCA)
- ✗ Do not make assumptions about a person's best interest based solely on their age, race, health or behaviour. Apart from being a poor way to determine a person's best interest it is also a form of discrimination which is against the law
- ✗ Do not make a decision without ALL of the relevant facts
- ✗ Do not make a decision on behalf of someone that may prejudice their future position if they later regain their mental capacity to make their own decision
- ✗ Do not make a decision based on what is convenient for the decision maker – such as removing life support if the decision maker desires the person's death

Sometimes a person's mental capacity is so affected that for the safety of themselves and others it is necessary to restrict that person's freedom or, in other words, deprive them of liberty. Under usual circumstances to deprive someone of their liberty is a violation of their human rights but, as long as the following two criteria are met, in some cases it is acceptable.

- It must be reasonably believed that it is necessary for the person to be restrained for their own safety or that of others
- The form of restraint must be proportionate to the risk of the person causing harm and the type of harm they are likely to cause

The Mental Capacity Act has provisions to detain people if the above two criteria are met. These are called "Deprivation of Liberty Safeguards" and they provide an extra level of protection for vulnerable people with reduced mental capacity. These safeguards can only be used if the person will be deprived of their liberty in a care home or hospital. In other settings the Court of Protection can authorise a deprivation of liberty.

Unnecessary or excessive restraint is an offense and could be liable to civil or criminal prosecution.

As previously discussed in this text, people with diminished mental capacity require extra safeguards but in particular relation to deprivation of liberty this action must be in the least restrictive way possible regardless of their age, ability or infirmity. The need to detain people while rare may be required in someone with profound learning difficulties or dementia, say. Also, as previously discussed, in spite of the fact that someone's liberty has been restricted they should still be cared for in ways that will continue to promote as much independence and choice while still ensuring their wellbeing.

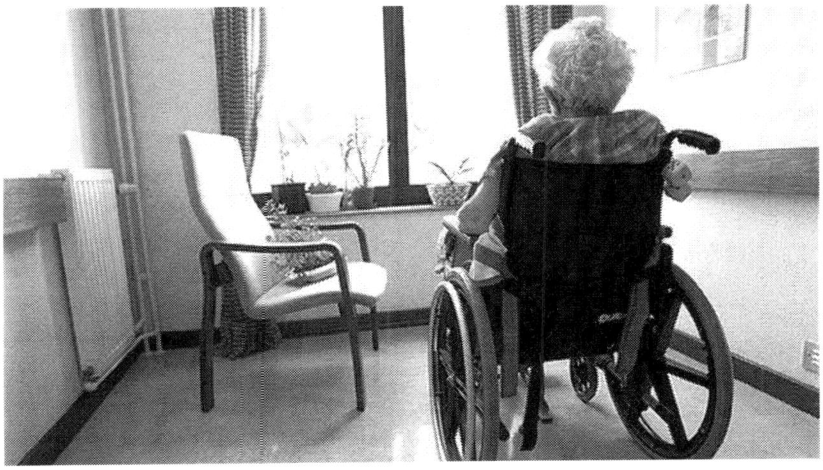

Proportional means…

As already stated, each case will need to be assessed individually but the outcome of the assessment and any subsequent actions must be in proportion to the situation. For instance the following actions may be appropriate for a person with advanced Alzheimer's but not for someone with learning difficulties

- The use of locks or key pads which stop a person leaving the building if they are prone to wonder off and get lost
- The use of medication which helps to calm the person and is prescribed by a doctor
- Close supervision
- Removing items from a person which could cause them harm

Care providers don't have to be experts about what is and is not a deprivation of liberty. They just need to know when a person might be deprived of their liberty and be prepared to take action if necessary.

When care providers are putting together the care plans of persons who are unable to consent to their care, they should consider whether any restrictions or restraint being proposed in the best interests of the person amount to a deprivation of liberty.

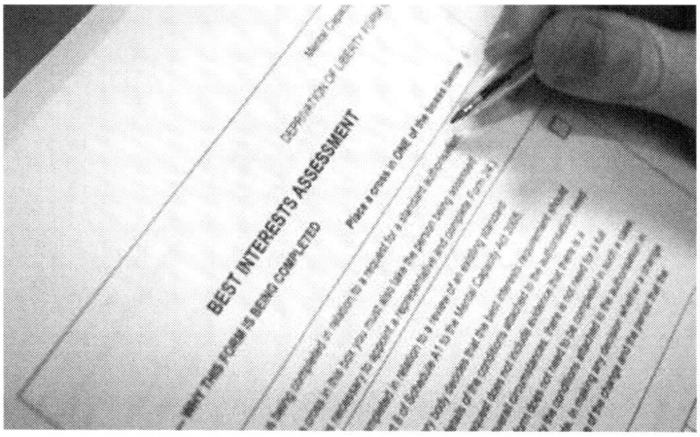

When it has been decided that it is in a person's best interest for their liberty to be restricted there are some key points to remember:

1. Decisions must not be arbitrary and should be a last resort
2. The same five principles which apply under the Mental Capacity Act still apply and must be adhered to strictly.
3. Any action must be in the best interest of the person
4. A person has the right to challenge the decision and request an IMCA

Authorising Deprivation of Liberty

The Deprivation of Liberty Safeguards (the Safeguards) can only apply to people who are in a care home or hospital. This includes where there are plans to move a person to a care home or hospital where they may be deprived of their liberty. Accordingly the care home or hospital is called the "managing authority". Only a "supervisory body" such as a local authority can authorise any form of deprivation of liberty.

An application can be made by a managing authority up to 28 days in advance of when it is needed. A supervisory body then appoints assessors to see if the conditions are met to allow the person to be deprived of their liberty under the safeguards.

The conditions include:

- The person is 18 or over (different safeguards apply for children).
- The person is suffering from a mental disorder.
- The person lacks capacity to decide for themselves about the restrictions which are proposed so they can receive the necessary care and treatment.
- The restrictions would deprive the person of their liberty.
- The proposed restrictions would be in the person's best interests.
- Whether the person should instead be considered for detention under the Mental Health Act.
- There is no valid advance decision to refuse treatment or support that would be overridden by any Safeguards process.

Only if all of the conditions met can deprivation of liberty be authorised. This may mean that the care home or hospital has to change its care plan so that the person can be supported in a less restrictive way and the supervisory body may put restrictions on the authorisation which the managing authority must follow. Further, the restrictions should stop as soon as they are no longer required without having to wait until the authorisation is finished.

On the other hand, authorisations cannot be extended. If it is felt that a person still needs to be deprived of their liberty at the end of an authorisation, the managing authority must request another standard authorisation.

If a care/nursing home or hospital makes an application to a local authority for a deprivation of liberty authorisation, it must inform the Care Quality Commission, once the outcome of the application is known. CQC provides a form for this purpose.

If a person subject to a deprivation of liberty authorisation should die while subject to the authorisation the local Coroner's Office should be informed by the care provider.

Urgent Applications

Occasionally there may be an urgent need to deprive someone of their liberty due to a sudden decline in their condition or recent extreme behaviour. In these situations the managing authority can use an urgent authorisation which it grants itself. The supervisory body will still need to be informed and, if necessary, an application for a standard authorisation will need to be commenced.

Before granting an urgent authorisation, the managing authority should try to speak to the family, friends and carers of the person. Their knowledge of the person could mean that deprivation of liberty can be avoided. The managing authority should make a record of their efforts to consult others.

The Safeguards

The primary safeguard in the assessment process is that at least two independent assessors (who must have received training for their role) will carry out the assessment. There will always be one mental health assessor and one best-interests assessor who will stop deprivation of liberty being authorised if they do not think all the conditions are met.

Secondly family, friends and paid carers who know the person well should be consulted as part of the assessment process. They may have suggestions about how the person can be supported without having to deprive them of their liberty. Those people who don't have family or friends who can represent them have a right to the support of an Independent Mental Capacity Advocate (IMCA) during the assessment process.

If the person has an unpaid relevant person's representative, both they and their representative are entitled to the support of an IMCA.

Another safeguards is that at all times, the fifth principle of the Mental Capacity Act, that any decision made in a person's best interests must be the least restrictive of their rights and freedoms, should be borne in mind.

The following is a list of the remainder of the safeguards which are available:

- The person must be appointed a relevant person's representative as soon as possible. Usually this will be a family member or friend who agrees to take this role. If there is no one willing or able to take this role on an unpaid basis, the supervisory body must pay someone, such as an advocate, to do this.
- The person and their representative can require the authorisation to be reviewed at any time, to see whether the criteria to deprive the person of their liberty are still met, and if so whether any conditions need to change.

- The person and their relevant person's representative have a right to challenge the deprivation of liberty in the Court of Protection at any time.
- If the person has an unpaid relevant person's representative, both they and their representative are entitled to the support of an IMCA. It is good practice for supervisory bodies to arrange for an IMCA to explain their role directly to both when a new authorisation has been granted.
- The home or hospital should do all it reasonably can to explain to a detained person and their family what their rights of appeal are and give support.

When Deprivation of Liberty is Wrongly Applied

Sometimes "support" can cross the line into excessive or unnecessary deprivation of liberty. Each case must be considered on its own merits, but it is helpful to consider whether:

The person subject to continuous supervision and control?
and
The person free to leave?*

*The focus of this question should not be whether a person seems to want to leave, but on how those who support them would react if they did want to leave.

Examples of when the line is crossed include:

- Frequent use of sedation/medication to control behaviour
- Regular use of physical restraint to control behaviour to which the person or their family verbally or physically objects
- The person is confined to a particular part of the establishment in which they are being cared for
- Staff take all decisions on behalf of the person or force them to take medication
- The care home has prevented the person from seeing friends or family
- Leaving someone who is unable to get around on their own in a room unattended

Note: The Safeguards can only be used if a person is in hospital or a care home. If a person is living in another setting, including in supported living or their own home, it is still possible to deprive the person of their liberty in their best interests, via an application to the Court of Protection.

Probably the most important aspect of all the Acts discussed so far in this text, and the one thread that runs through them all, is the aim to keep vulnerable people safe, free from harm and respected as valued as an individual.

> ***"Abuse is a violation of an individual's human and civil rights by any other person or persons"***
> *(No Secrets Department of Health 2000)*

When a person's mental abilities deteriorate or when they become more dependent on others and less able to speak up for themselves they become vulnerable. This vulnerability can lead to abuse in the forms of emotional, financial or chemical abuse and may or may not be deliberate. There are usually indicators that this is going on and it is important that policies and procedures exist in every professional care situation to deal with it. Staff should be trained in recognizing the signs of abuse and how to report incidents of, or suspicions about, abuse taking place. The following is a list of signs that abuse may be occurring:

1. ***CHEMICAL ABUSE****; over-use of medication to control or manage their behaviour.*
   a. Constantly appearing drowsy
   b. Repeated falls
   c. Lack of medication reviews
2. ***EMOTIONAL ABUSE:*** *the use of threats or intimidation intended to cause fear or lower self- esteem*
   a. Anxiety, confusion or general resignation
   b. Extreme submissiveness or dependency in contrast with known capacity
   c. Sharp changes in behaviour in the presence of certain persons
   d. Excessive or inappropriate craving for attention
   e. Extreme self-abusive behaviour such as self-mutilation or head banging
3. ***FINANCIAL/MATERIAL ABUSE:*** *the extortion of money or manipulation in order to gain money or goods*
   a. Unexplained or sudden withdrawal of money from accounts
   b. Contrast between known income or capital and unnecessarily poor living conditions especially where it had developed recently
   c. Personal possessions of value go missing from the home without satisfactory explanation

These forms of abuse can also be the CAUSE of the reduction in mental capacity.
Vigilance for the signs is vital!
Report them immediately to the manager, local authority or even the police!

As serious as the act of abuse is the act of neglect. Again, neglect can be intentional or unintentional and there are many signs that it is occurring such as unkempt clothing or belongings, loss of weight, poor hygiene or untreated injuries. But neglect can also occur in the form of not fulfilling the emotional wellbeing of the individual or violating their rights. Making a decision for someone without due consideration to their wishes or to the implications of the decision is a neglect of duty. Carers, advocates and those appointed to look after the person all have a clearly defined duty of care under the law and a breach of this duty is as serious as physical abuse and potentially punishable by a fine or even imprisonment.

People acting on behalf of someone else must fully understand their role and carry out their duties to the best of their ability.

More information can be found in our *Safeguarding Vulnerable Adults (04SV)* text.

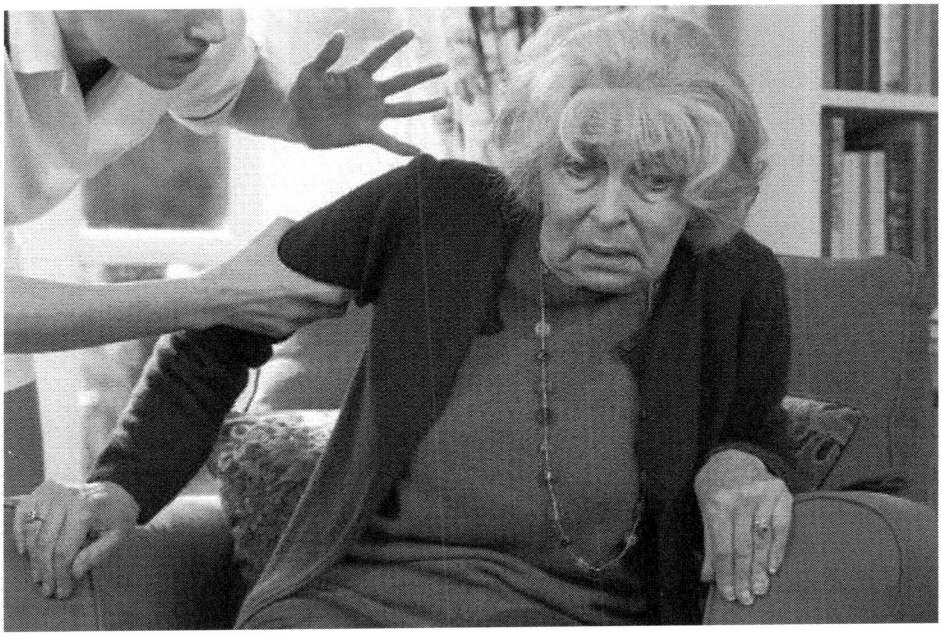

It is helpful for people whose mental capacity is declining to maintain a sense of normality for as long as possible. This will help the person to feel independent and maintain their self-esteem.[1] When they feel safe and secure in their environment and lifestyle it is easier for someone to make decisions about what it is that they want to do.

The ways this can be done include:

- Support the person in writing notes of the things that they want to remember.
- Pin a weekly timetable to the wall.
- "A place for everything and everything in its place" – ALL THE TIME
- Have a daily newspaper delivered to prompt the resident to look at the date.
- Put labels on cupboards and drawers.
- Write reminders and put them in places where the person will see them.
- Picture symbols can be equally as effective i.e. picture of toilet/shower.
- Put up pictures of familiar family and friends around their living space.
- Let them bring familiar bedding and furnishings.
- Encourage them to choose their own new clothes
- Many watches and phones have alarms that can act as reminders.
- Install safety devices such as smoke/heat/gas detectors.

Not all of these techniques will work for everyone, some may even increase confusion. Trial and error is the best way to determine what works

Next, there are steps that a carer can take to assist the decision making process:

1. Assume the person has the capability of making the decision
2. Encourage them to make the decision themselves
3. Ensure they have and understand all the relevant information (this may mean going over the information several times or presenting it in a different way)
4. Ensure they understand the alternatives and the consequences of any decision
5. Suggest they choose a time and place where they are most able to make a decision
6. Enlist the help of others if necessary

Remember that simply making a bad decision is not proof that a person lacks the mental capacity to make a decision

[1] Source: Alzheimers.org.uk

INVOLVEMENT IN CARE PLANNING

There are often cases when someone knows well in advance that they will at some point have reduced mental capacity. Others may look forward and wish to make plans “just in case”. The Mental Capacity Acts have provision for people to plan for the future time when they may be in a position of reduced capacity, while still ensuring that decisions they made while they had a full complement of capacity are respected and obeyed.

Wherever possible, including the person in discussion about their care should be the highest priority. There are three key reasons for this: it is a fundamental part of the Person-Centred Approach (to be discussed in more detail later in this text), it is key to ensuring them that their best interests are the priority, and it is the best way for the individual to retain as much control over their life quality as possible. It is also a good idea to include people who know the person well as a person may not have the same perception of their needs as those around them.

For instance if a person usually reads The Times newspaper every morning they would appreciate having a copy available to read each day, and this will promote individuality and mental stimulation. Involving the client in discussions about their care package will help the carer to find out small things that may mean a lot to the client and allow the carer to include them in their daily routine.

***REMEMBER** - Regular reviewing of assessments will be a vital part of the role of the carer.*

Assessments and reviews will be required when:

There is change in a person’s physical or mental health

The person requests a review

When a review is requested by significant others, such as family and social worker

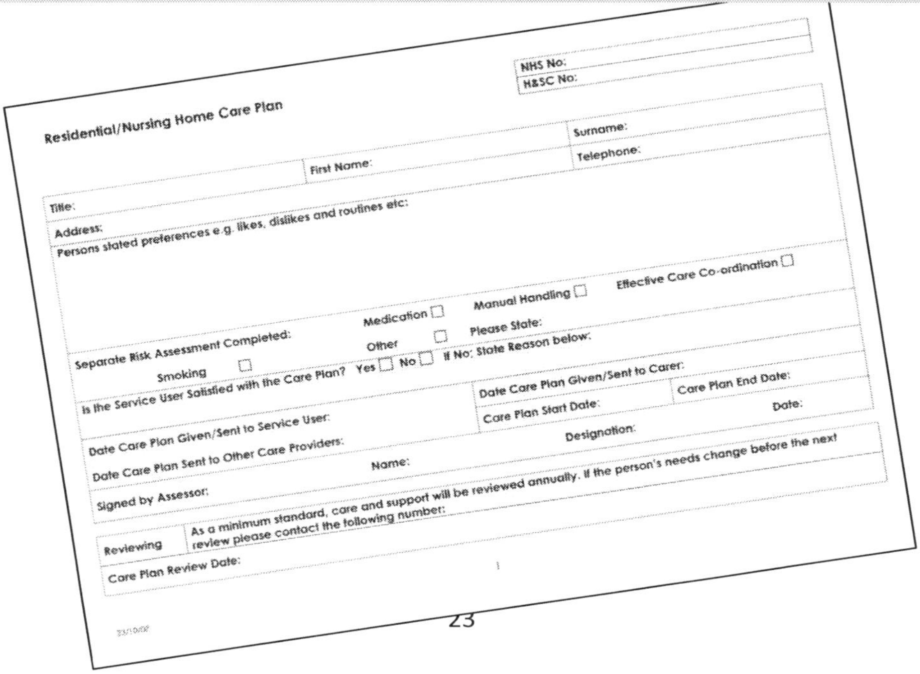

NHS No:
H&SC No:

Residential/Nursing Home Care Plan

Surname:
First Name: Telephone:
Title:
Address:
Persons stated preferences e.g. likes, dislikes and routines etc:

Separate Risk Assessment Completed: Medication ☐ Manual Handling ☐ Effective Care Co-ordination ☐
Smoking ☐ Other ☐ Please State:
Is the Service User Satisfied with the Care Plan? Yes ☐ No ☐ If No: State Reason below:
Date Care Plan Given/Sent to Service User: Date Care Plan Given/Sent to Carer:
Care Plan Start Date: Care Plan End Date:
Date Care Plan Sent to Other Care Providers:
Signed by Assessor: Name: Designation: Date:
Reviewing: As a minimum standard, care and support will be reviewed annually. If the person's needs change before the next review please contact the following number:
Care Plan Review Date:

As part already discussed some people may be aware that their mental capacity will be diminished in the future (or just wish to prepare for the worst) and in these cases it is a good idea to lay out clearly a person's wishes for the future, even the parts that are unpleasant to think about, before they are no longer able to do so. Often questions about how to handle End of Life Care are put to people upon admission to a care home. This may feel awkward or inappropriate for both parties but this is the best time to look at these options as the person is likely to be in the best position, medically.

The NHS recommends making an "Advance Statement"[2]. This is a statement where a person may put down in writing their preferences, wishes, beliefs and values regarding future care, as well as things they particularly do not want to happen.

There are several points to consider:

- What are the patient's spiritual or religious beliefs and how would they like them to be enacted?
- Where would they like to be cared for – a hospital, a nursing home, a hospice, or at home?
- Are there any practical requests such as a shower instead of a bath, sleeping with the window open?
- Is there anything that they would specifically not wish to happen, such as any medical procedure they would refuse?
- Have they got a will, insurance policy or bank accounts that people need to know about?

These statements need to be as detailed as the service user requires and could even include details such as what flowers they would like at their funeral. Having a plan in place, via this statement, not only makes things easier for the family members but also ensures that everyone is aware of the wishes of the service user in the event they are no longer able to communicate them.

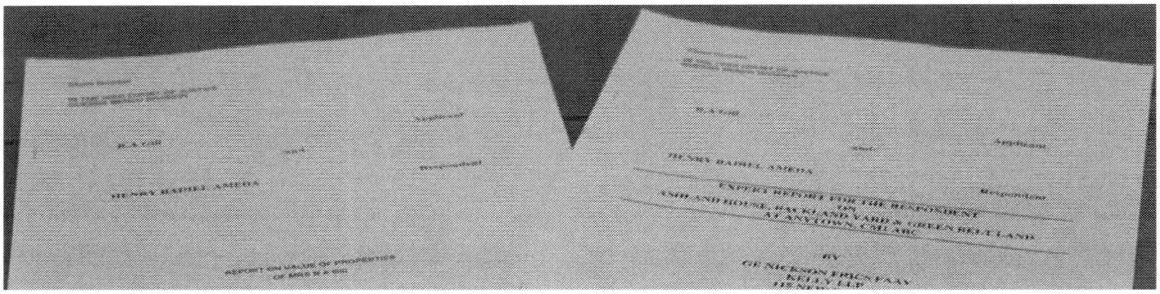

[2] Source: NHS.UK

Advance Care Planning (ACP), Advanced Directives and Advanced Decisions are all other terms for a living will which is a decision you can make now to refuse specific treatments in the future. Unlike the Advanced Statements discussed in the previous section, which are expressions of wishes to be fulfilled in as much as they are possible, a living will is legally binding as long as it is correctly codified and doctors are obliged to comply with its instructions.

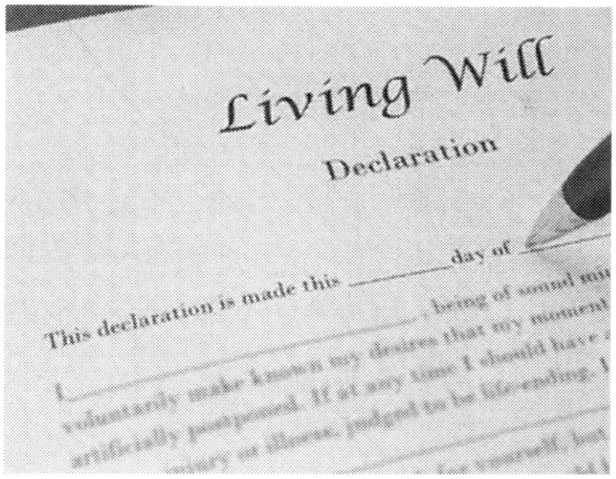

Planning for possible health care decisions that may arise in the future, particularly those that arise when a services user is not fully capable of expressing their own wishes, may seem excessive. In fairness, not everyone will feel the need to set in place any special arrangements. However, if it becomes apparent that someone may suffer a reduction in mental capacity in the future it is important to raise the topic and give the person an opportunity to consider their feelings about such an occurrence.

If the individual feels that there are things they wish to raise then it is important to review their choices and involve, in as much as requested by the service user, their family, medical specialists and social care professionals. This discussion may lead to a living will being drawn up reflecting their choices, with the aim that decisions in certain situations have already been made, relieving the family of having to take these decisions and what is already a difficult time. It is key to remember that a living will is not a one off event and should be reviewed, by all parties concerned, from time to time.

Again, as required under The Mental Capacity Act 2005 a carer should support the individual as much as possible to make their own decision. It is also a legal requirement that any living will be taken into account both when assessing the individual's needs and planning their care package. It is important to understand the obligations under the law for two reasons:

- The wishes and dignity of the service users should be of the highest priority. They have the right to refuse any treatment, including resuscitation, if they so desire.
- However, if a person's mental capacity is not properly assessed or is mishandled there could be very serious legal implications.

If a carer is unsure about anything to do with a Living Will, they should speak to their manager who may ask the help of professionals, such as a doctor or a lawyer, if required. Alternatively, more information can be found out about this at GOV.UK

In spite of the two previous sections there may be times when an individual is not "capable" of giving consent to their medication or treatment and there is no indication as to their wishes. This can be particularly difficult for the carer as they are generally the person responsible for administering the medication to the person. Situations such as these are covered under the guidelines of the Mental Capacity Act 2005, allowing decisions to be made on behalf of an individual if it is in their best interests. If the carer finds themselves in this position the guidelines in the act should be followed as shown below:

Balancing the Duty of Care with the Rights of the Individual
Often the person may disagree with decisions made on their behalf or will make decisions that put them at risk. For instance a dementia sufferer might want to go out alone without realising that they easily become disoriented and forgetful, or they might refuse to take their medication or to eat. In these instances, principals of the MCA will apply. The carer should ensure that they document any issues that need assessing, so that a full review of the situation can be held. If any action is taken it needs to be as unobtrusive and unrestrictive as practical.

Remember: Over-medication in people is a form of abuse. There are other ways of managing behaviour that should be explored first.

Guidance can also be found in the British Human Rights Act which extends the following rights to individuals to:

- be respected
- be treated equally and not be discriminated against
- be treated as an individual
- be treated in a dignified way
- privacy
- be protected from danger and harm
- communicate using their preferred methods of communication and language

ADVOCACY SERVICES

From time to time the person may require an independent advocate to speak on their behalf. This could be for any number of reasons including:

- To express the wishes of the person
- Where there is conflict between the individual and the informal carer
- Where the informal carer does not feel confident or able to speak
- Where the person is unable to access a service
- Where a professional feels that the persons expressed wishes have been influenced by others
- Where a person's views may need to be clarified, particularly when a decision to move into residential care is required
- If the person has been 'sectioned' under the Mental Health Act 1983

INDEPENDENT MENTAL CAPACITY ADVOCATE (IMCA)

The role of the IMCA was introduced by the Mental Capacity Act to further safeguard people who lack the capacity to independently make significant decisions about things such as where they live or serious medical treatment options and have no-one appropriate to speak for them.

An IMCA must be instructed for people in the following circumstances:

- Aged 16 or over
- A decision needs to be made about either a long-term change in accommodation or serious medical treatment (although it is sometimes required for Care Reviews or Adult Protection
- The person lacks capacity to make that decision
- There is no one independent of services, such as a family member or friend, who is "appropriate to consult" (in adult protection cases an IMCA may be instructed even where family members or others are available to be consulted)

IMCAs may also be appointed where there are gaps between appointments of person's representatives, where requested by the person, their representative, or if the Supervisory Body believes either could benefit from the support of an IMCA.

An IMCA cannot start to work for a person until they are instructed to do so by an "authorised" person, such as a social worker, care manager working for the local authority or hospital, appropriate medical professional or the chair of the adult protection proceedings or contact from the Supervisory body where deprivation of liberty is being considered. A carer could also speak to your local IMCA provider directly to ensure that an IMCA is instructed where required.

If a person is not eligible for the IMCA service but could benefit from the support of an advocate, a carer could find out what other advocacy services are available in the area. In England and Wales this information can be found from the Action for Advocacy database.

The Role of the IMCA

1. *Gathering Information:-*
    a. Meeting and interviewing (where possible) the person. The person may not be able to contribute much to such a meeting but it is still likely that the IMCA will want to meet them as it would be difficult for them to represent them without doing this. It is a legal right for an IMCA to meet with the person but it is also important that the IMCA maintain as much privacy and confidentiality as possible at this meeting so the person feels they can talk freely. Examine relevant health and social care records
    b. Get the views of professionals and paid workers. Health and social care staff are an important source of information for an IMCA. Knowledge of the person can help ensure the right decisions are made. Carers should feel confident to share information with the IMCA such as their views and beliefs and the relationships they have with others, as well as advice such as how best to communicate with the person, what support they need
    c. Get the views of anybody else who can give information about the wishes and feelings, beliefs or values of the person.
    d. Find out other information which may be relevant to the decision. One of the legal powers of IMCAs is to be able to look at and take copies of relevant records. This includes health records, records held by local authorities and records held by care homes (such as care assessments and plans, daily log books, or staff rotas to check levels of support available). If records requested by an IMCA do not seem to be relevant to the decision, however, they would have to justify their reasons for withholding them.

2. *Evaluating information:-*
    a. Check that the person has been supported to be involved in the decision.
    b. Try to work out what the person's wishes and feelings would be if they had capacity to make the decision and what values and beliefs would influence this.
    c. Make sure that different options have been considered.
    d. Decide whether to ask for a second medical opinion where it is a serious medical treatment decision.

3. *Making representations:-*
    a. IMCAs should raise any issues and concerns with the decision maker. This could be done verbally or in writing.
    b. IMCAs are required to produce a report for the person who instructed them. In most cases this should be provided to the decision maker before the decision is made.
    c. People who instruct IMCAs must pay attention to any issues raised by the IMCA in making their decision.

4. *Challenging decisions*
    a. In many cases IMCAs will be able to resolve any concerns they have with the decision maker before the decision is made. Where this has not been possible IMCAs may formally challenge the decision-making process. They can use local complaint procedures or try to get the matter looked at by the Court of Protection.

Note - When the IMCA asks you to meet the person the following information would be helpful to them:

- How best to help the person to communicate?
- Whether there are times of the day when the person might find this easier?
- Whether there are any risks the IMCA should be aware of. For example, the person might be physically violent or have a history of making false allegations.

The IMCA must not be expected to take on any supervision or support roles that are normally undertaken by staff. For example, if the person needs to be supervised continuously it would not be acceptable for the IMCA to meet the person without other staff present.

HELP FOR THOSE WORKING IN THE CARE INDUSTRY

One of the surprising aspects of the Mental Capacity Act is that it provides a level of protection for workers in the care industry and people making decisions on behalf of others. As long as a decision maker does everything in their power to comply with the requirements of the law they will be safe from prosecution. In particular this means (as summarised from the text so far):

1. Complying with The 5 Principles
2. Carrying out a proper and reasonable assessment of the person's capability
3. Taking reasonable actions which are in the best interest of the individual being looked after.
4. Clearly and concisely recording details of the decision making process and the end result in order to demonstrate compliance with the law

No matter whether the decision is big or small, whether it has no effect or a dramatic, long lasting and irreversible effect, as long as the decision maker has taken due care, given the decision full consideration and followed the above guidelines, they will be safe from any repercussions under the law.

There may be times when an urgent decision is required but, again, providing as much care as possible is taken and the decision is made in the best interests of the individual to the extent that is possible under the circumstances, then the law will still apply.

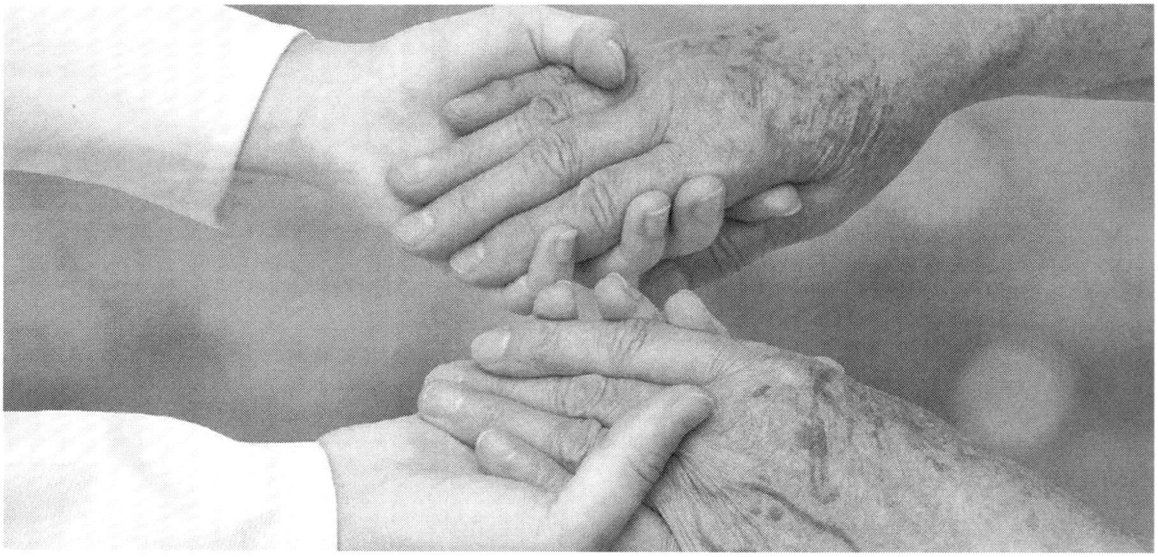

PERSON TO PERSON CARE

With the best will in the world carers may be unaware that their actions have a negative impact on a person with reduced mental capacity. The best way to avoid this is to:

See the person first not the condition.

People often make assumptions that people with reduced mental capacity cannot make good choices and should be treated like babies. These are very degrading and dangerous stereotypes.

When caring for people with reduced mental capacity:

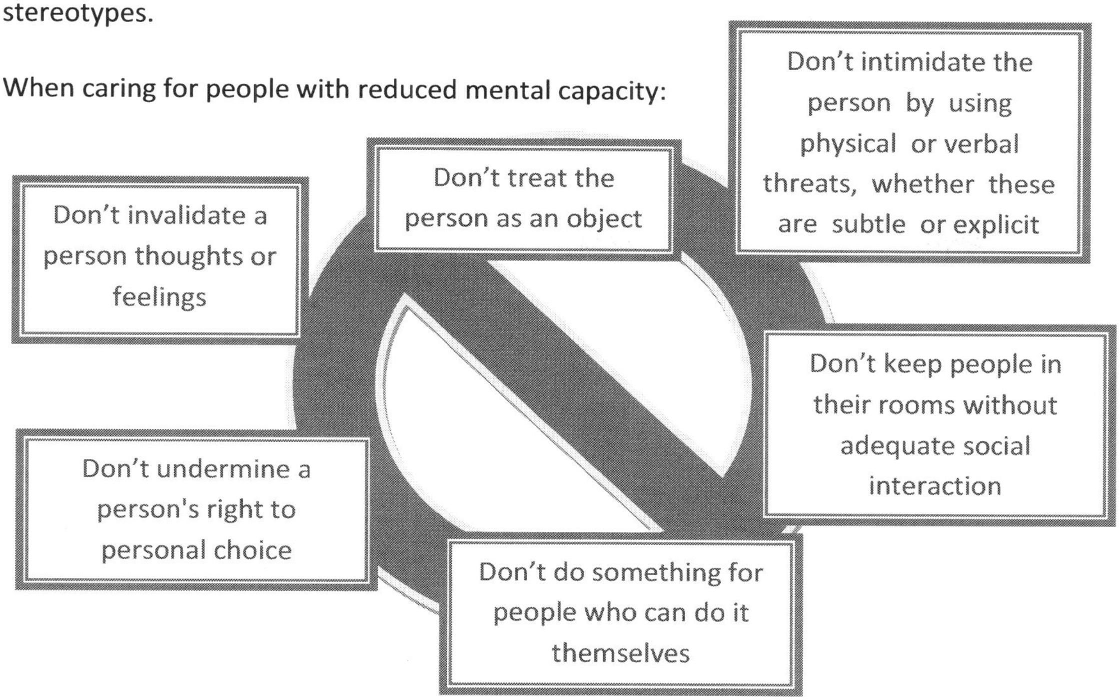

Having a negative effect on a person with reduced capacity and may even make their mental state worse by deskilling and devaluing them. It is as though the care is done **to** them and not **for** them and reduces their power of self-determination, a basic human right.

Instead the role of a carer should be to provide:

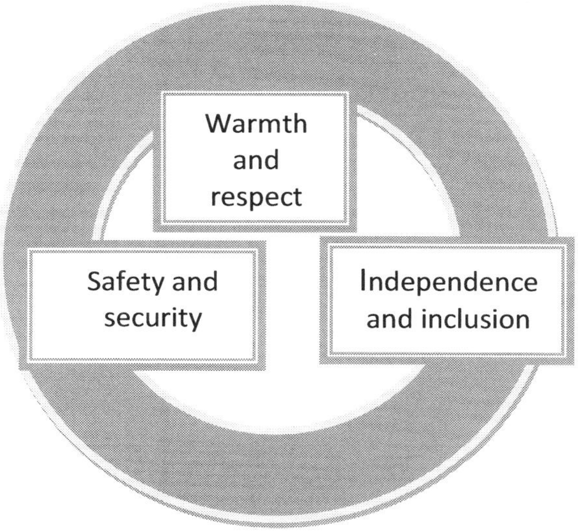

EFFECTIVE COMMUNICATION

A person will have no control over their condition or the corresponding reduction in mental capacity. As the condition progresses the ability to communicate deteriorates and yet the person can have even more complex communication needs, meaning their need to communicate increases. So it up to the carer to ensure that communication with the individual is effective. This means that it is the carer who must change the way that they communicate in order to meet the person's needs. While it is not possible to overcome all difficulties a person may have there are several techniques that can help with most situations.

This further reinforces the need for person-to-person care, where the carer can rely on other forms of communication to understand what the person is trying to communicate i.e. body language, facial expression and behaviour. In fact, when a person's language skills become impaired they rely more on their other senses such as sight and touch so visual cues can be very useful.

Care plans need to be kept up to date with the current "best way" to communicate with the person. As communication becomes increasingly difficult it may be helpful to:

- Make sure the person's sight and hearing are not impaired. It might be a faulty hearing aid or the wrong glasses prescription that is causing the problem
- Speak slowly, clearly, face to face and at eye level.
- Where appropriate, show warmth and sensitivity through touch, i.e. a simple hold of the hand or arm. Professional carers should not act like robots, and although care should be taken not to overstep boundaries or invade personal space, at times a little hug can show empathy and understanding.
- Pay attention to a person's body language. Often people whose language is impaired will communicate through non-verbal means.

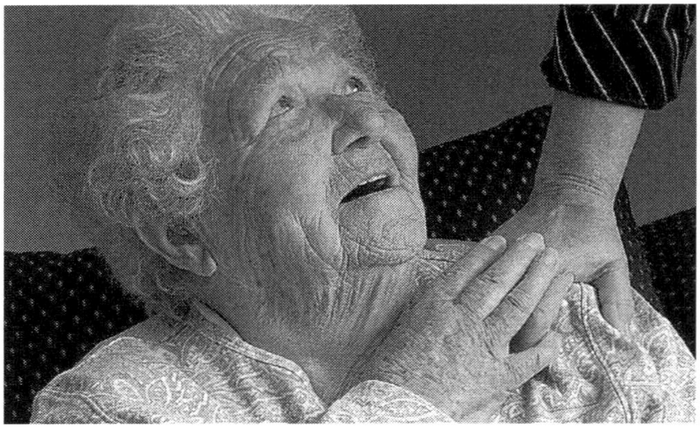

- Be aware of your own body language.
- Find out what combination of word reminders / prompting words, guidance and demonstration is needed to communicate effectively with the person.
- Always try to gain the persons attention before speaking.

SUPPORT NETWORKS AND ORGANISATIONS

Loss of mental capacity is difficult for the sufferer and their friends and family alike. If the carer feels that they, the person or their friends and family need extra help or advice this can be found from the following places:

- The individuals G.P. can refer for counselling
- Social Services will provide support for both the sufferer and the family
- Care home manager or key worker
- The Alzheimer's Society or Age UK
- Local carers groups
- Domiciliary services
- Benefits agencies
- Respite services
- NHS Direct

Leading the fight against dementia
Alzheimer's Society

NHS Direct
CALL 111
when it's less urgent than 999

age UK
The new force combining
Age Concern and Help the Aged

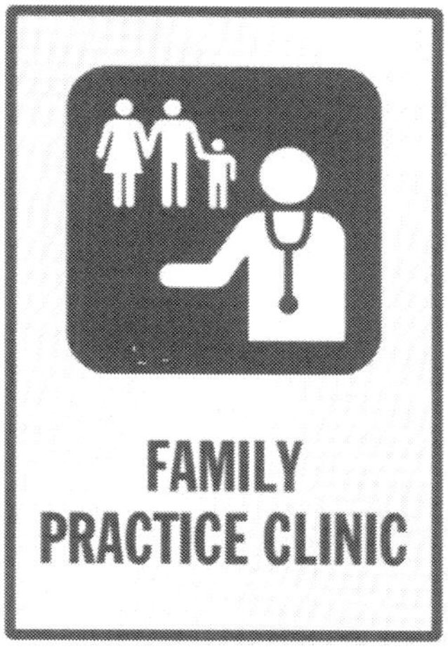

ROLES AND RESPONSIBILITIES OF THE CARER

As can be seen below there are many people involved in the care of vulnerable elderly people but the person requiring care must be at the centre of the circle in accordance with the current Person-Centred approach to care and for the best outcomes for the person. The outside ring represents the connection these people have with each other as well as the person in need of care.

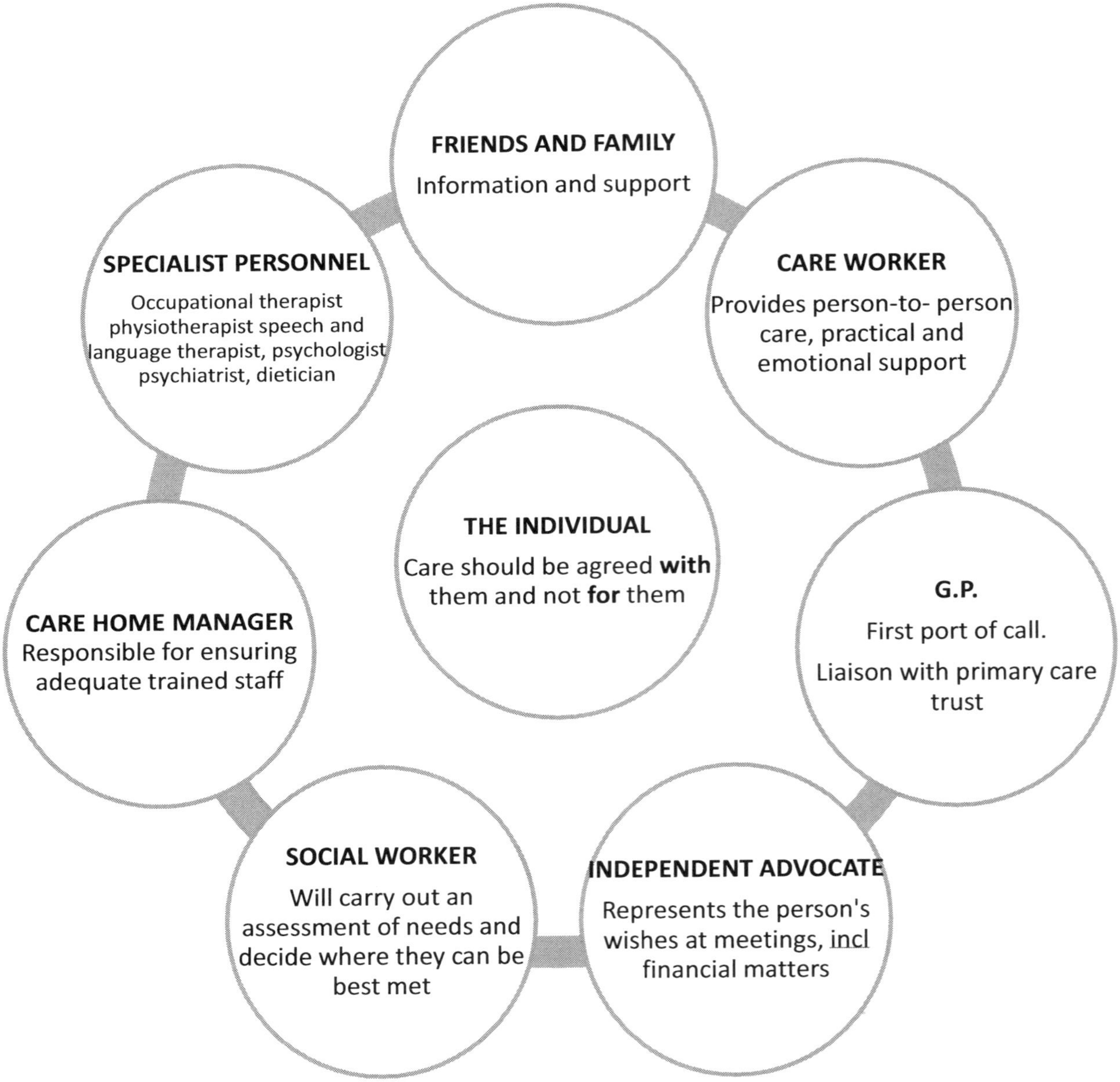

EFFECTIVE RECORDING

Keeping accurate and up to date records about a person is essential and an integral part of the carer's role. It is important for monitoring both the progress of their condition as well as the overall health and well-being. Mental capacity can change rapidly and the changes must not only be communicated among all the people involved in the care but also having a detailed record will assist if the sufferer becomes incapable of communicating their wishes at any point.

Everyone, including informal carers, must be strongly encouraged to ensure records are kept in a detailed, timely and accurate way as working together as a team is the only way to ensure proper care is provided and good communication is at the heart of any team work.

Setting up suitable procedures can assist in ensuring excellent record keeping. Instructions on how to remain objective (avoid bias or personal opinions), when and how records should be taken, and what to include, should be made clear to everyone who has dealings with the person.

COMMON PROBLEMS WITH RECORDING TO WATCH OUT FOR

- Inappropriate language
- Lack of confidentiality
- Irrelevance
- Lack of objectivity
- Not fact based
- Not succinct (too long)
- Poor format
- Not written for sharing (code words etc)
- Not used as an analysis tool
- Illegible (poor handwriting)
- Not Person-Centred
- Lack of user involvement
- Disrespect to a person
- Focus on negatives

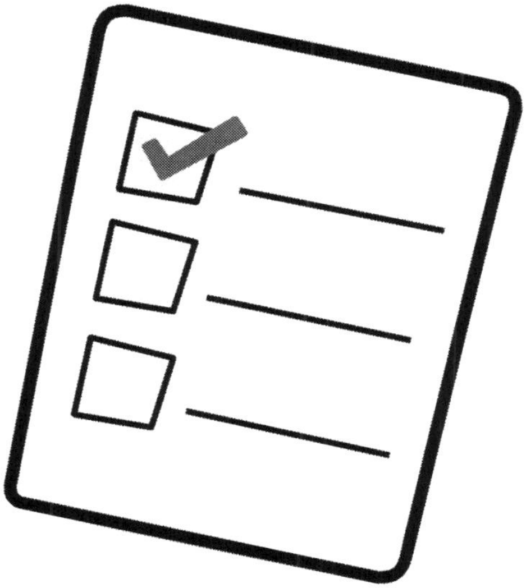

The best solution for all of these issues is to always remember the reason that the records are being kept:
TO PROVIDE THE BEST CARE POSSIBLE FOR THE INDIVIDUAL CONCERNED.

POLICIES AND PROCEDURES

The Procedures and Policies of a care home should be carefully prepared to ensure they are practical and useful, they should be effectively communicated to both staff and service users and they should be reviewed from time to time to ensure they are kept up to date and adapted when needed. Staff need to ensure that they familiarise themselves with the policies and procedures BEFORE dealing with any clients and that they are informed of any changes that occur subsequently.

P&Ps help carers in their daily tasks because it lets them:

- ✓ know what to expect and what is expected of them
- ✓ know what to do when certain events arise
- ✓ know where to go to find out more
- ✓ have a effective guide for working alongside clients and their families
- ✓ provide guidance when faced with an ethical dilemma

If carers are not aware of an organisations policies and procedures, or choose to disregard them, they run the risk of:

- ✗ Working differently to everyone else and therefore not working as a team
- ✗ Not using safe systems at work and as a consequence putting themselves and the individual they care for at risk
- ✗ Not knowing or helping to achieve organizational objectives
- ✗ Appearing unprofessional or presenting the organization in an unprofessional way

We will never know when we might be in a position of reduced metal capacity. It can happen to anyone at any time for any reason and it can last just a short while or the rest of our lives. When we have lost our capacity to make decisions about our lives, however, that makes us vulnerable but that does not mean we have lost our rights as human beings. We still have the right to be respected, to be treated fairly, and above all to decide how we want to live our lives in as much extent as possible.

In order to protect these moral rights, many Acts of Parliament and other Safeguards have been put into place to help preserve these but also ensure we are looked after in the best way possible. Though this issue is highly complex we hope that the information provided in this text has gone some way to explain how to act in someone's best interests (as well as why this is important), how to safeguard someone from harm and how to promote as independent a life as possible. We also hope that we have shown how it may be possible to inadvertently deprive someone of their liberty unnecessarily as well as how to spot when someone else is doing so out of cruelty or convenience, as well as what to do when it occurs.

Everyone has the right to live a happy and fulfilled life, regardless of their mental capacity and no-one has the right to take away a person's dignity by removing their right to make decisions about their life.

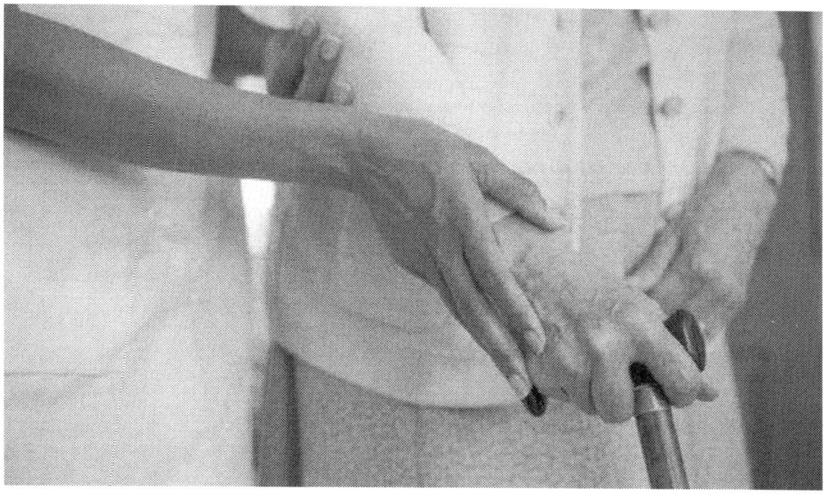

OTHER RELEVANT LEGISLATION

HEALTH AND SOCIAL CARE ACT 2012

This act forms an umbrella under which all vulnerable people in whatever care setting are protected. It replaces the previous CARE STANDARDS ACT 2000 (which replaced the Registered Homes Act 1984) and the HEALTH ACT 1999. The Act follows the National Care Standards Commission (NCSC) which later became the Commission for Social Care Inspection (CSCI) and now is the Care Quality Commission (CQC)

The government introduced National Minimum Standards and established the General Social Care Council (GSCC) for England and the Care Council for Wales. These work towards raising the standards of practice through codes of conduct and practice. The Act requires that any agency supplying care to a person within their own home (domiciliary) must be registered.

NATIONAL SERVICE FRAMEWORK FOR OLDER PEOPLE

A National Service Framework (NSF) for older people (aged over 55) was published by the Department of Health in 2001. It is a 10 year framework for improving the health and social care of older people in England.

DATA PROTECTION ACT 1998

This act governs the storage and processing of personal data held in manual records and on computers. Under this act, rights are protected by forcing organizations to follow proper and sound practices, known as data protection principles (DPP).

The data protection Act contains 8 principles which state that all data must be;

1. Processed fairly and lawfully
2. Obtained and used only for specified and lawful purposes
3. Adequate, relevant and not excessive
4. Accurate, and where necessary, kept up to date
5. Kept for no longer than necessary
6. Processed in accordance with the individuals rights
7. Kept secure
8. Transferred only to countries that offer adequate data protection

NHS AND COMMUNITY CARE ACT 1990

Requires social services to assess an individual's needs for living within the community. They should also provide clear procedures for complaints, comments, and registration and inspection requirements. Reviews of a person's ability to contribute should also be taken into consideration.

THE HEALTH AND SAFETY ACT 1974

Requires the employer and the employee to take responsibility for health and safety whilst carrying out work. The act requires employers to provide a safe working environment and supply any equipment required to carry out the role i.e. personal protective equipment.

LEARN CARE EXCEL

Matthews House
21 Thorley Park Road
Bishops Stortford
CM23 3NG

Tel: 07774 880880

info@learncareexcel.co.uk
www.learncareexcel.co.uk

Printed in Great Britain
by Amazon

33320411R00024